Learning through SBAs:
220 Single best answers for medical school finals

Dr Elliott Lever

Preface

Preparing for finals needs to combine question practice, with detailed and broad knowledge. This book aims to help your work towards your exams. The range of difficulty of the questions is skewed to the harder end of the spectrum. Each question aims to provide at least one learning point more than just doing an SBA question. There are simple 1 step questions for checking knowledge.

Wishing you the best in your preparation and future success.

Table of Contents

1. Respiratory

1. A central lung lesion on CT thorax is most likely to be indicative of a

A. squamous cell carcinoma
B. adenocarcinoma
C. small cell carcinoma
D. undifferentiated
E. large cell carcinoma

2. The type of lung cancer most commonly found to cause hypercalcaemia is

A. squamous cell carcinoma
B. adenocarcinoma
C. small cell carcinoma
D. undifferentiated
E. large cell carcinoma

3. A 60 year old has a restrictive pattern on spirometry and is anti-Jo positive. Considering the likely underlying diagnosis which physical sign may be present?

A. splinter haemorrhages
B. malar rash
C. Gottron's papules
D. pretibial ulceration
E. erythema multiforme

4. A 59 year old is admitted with pneumonia. Which of the following results is most suggestive of an empyema?

A. pleural fluid protein 12g/L
B. pleural fluid pH 6.9
C. pleural fluid glucose
D. pleural fluid LDH to serum LDH ratio of 0.7

E.   pleural fluid protein to serum protein ratio of 0.6

5. A nurse asks you what the oxygen levels should be for a patient who has had recent BIPAP

A.   saturations 94-98%
B.   saturations 85%+
C.   saturations 88-92%
D.   Po2 of 10 regardless of saturations
E.   Po2 of 9 regardless of saturations

6. A right sided effusion was aspirated. Pleural fluid analysis was in keeping with an exudate. Out of the following which is a potential cause?

A.   tuberculosis
B.   heart failure
C.   hypoalbuminaemia
D.   liver failure
E.   renal failure

7. A 54 year old with a recent exacerbation of asthma is referred to clinic. She had a recent course of prednisolone which has now finished. She has had 5 exacerbations in last 6 months and is currently taking her salbutamol I4 times a day and takes inhaled corticosteroid.
The next step in managing the asthma is to add in

A.   montelukast
B.   oral prednisolone
C.   long acting beta-agonist inhaler
D.   increase dose inhaled corticosteroids
E.   oral theophylline

8. A 70 year old man presents with nasal crusting, nose bleeds and joint pains. What is the most likely abnormality on chest x ray?

A.   fibrosis
B.   effusion
C.   nodules

D. hilar lymphadenopathy
E. apical shadowing

9. The following cause a lower zone pattern of pulmonary fibrosis apart from

A. idiopathic pulmonary fibrosis
B. silicosis
C. rheumatoid arthritis
D. scleroderma
E. methotrexate

10. Which of these statements regarding TB are false?

A. latent TB is treated with a course of 3 months of anti-TB medication
B. Mantoux testing is done routinely to diagnose TB
C. the IRIS syndrome is treated with steroids
D. evidence of BCG in preventing extra-pulmonary TB is lacking
E. directly observed therapy is used in cases of TB

11. A 70 year old man is treated for pneumonia which is cavitating and is slow to improve. There are no positive cultures. Cavitating pneumonia is not generally an associated feature of this pathogen

A. Klebsiella
B. TB
C. Staphylococcus
D. Streptococcus species
E. M. Catarrhalis

12. The most common radiographic feature seen on CXR in a case of PE is

A. an area of oligaemia
B. pleural effusion
C. consolidation
D. juxtapleural opacity
E. no focal abnormality

13. Which of the following indicate a need for BIPAP?

A.   pH 7.36 Pco2 5.0 Po2 9.0 Hco3 23 lactate 1.5
B.   pH 7.30 Pco2 9.0 Po2 8.2 Hco3 26 lactate 1.7
C.   pH 7.26 Pco2 3.5 Po2 8.0 Hco3 15 lactate 3.0
D.   pH 7.40 Pco2 9.0 Po2 7.5 Hco3 36 lactate 1.0
E.   pH 7.56 Pco2 3.0 Po2 25.0 Hco3 32 lactate 2.5

14. An 89 year old is admitted with an exacerbation of COPD. GCS is 7. CXR shows no focal consolidation. Relative contraindications for BIPAP apart from

A.   undrained pneumothorax
B.   reduced GCS
C.   inability to consent
D.   pneumonia
E.   confusion

15. A patient has a DVT diagnosed and during the admission had a significant upper GI bleed that was successfully treated endoscopically. Appropriate management should be

A.   aspirin
B.   treatment dalteparin
C.   warfarin
D.   IVC filter
E.   intravenous heparin

16. A patient is admitted with tachypnoea and wheeze. Blood gases on air are pH 7.38, PC02 6.8 pO2 8.2 HCO3 33 lactate 1.0. These blood gases show

A.   type 1 respiratory failure
B.   type 2 respiratory failure
C.   type 2 respiratory failure (chronic)
D.   metabolic alkalosis
E.   respiratory alkalosis

17. A 60 year old with severe COPD presents with breathlessness over the last 6 hours. He has had a chronic nonproductive cough. There is globally reduced air entry and his saturations are 80% on room air. HR 130 BP 115/70 Temp 36.5C
The first part of his initial management should be

A. Nebs
B. BIPAP
C. antibiotics
D. IV fluids
E. steroids

18. A 73 year old woman with emphysema is admitted with pleuritic chest pain. To exclude a PE the most appropriate test is

A. ECHO
B. CTPA
C. MRI
D. V/Q scan
E. spirometry

19. A 19 year old had mild chest discomfort and came to accident and emergency. He is sitting comfortably saturating 98% on air. CXR showed a 4.5cm rim of air and no mediastinal shift. What is the most appropriate action?

A. drain
B. urgent insertion of a cannula into the 2nd intercostal space
C. aspiration
D. oxygen and observation
E. discharge with follow-up by the respiratory clinic

20. Life-threatening asthma features include all apart from

A. PEF<33%
B. sats <92%
C. low Pco2
D. cyanosis
E. hypotension

21. A patient is severely unwell with high oxygen requirements. CT chest is in keeping with pulmonary haemorrhages. Which autoantibody is found in this condition?

A.   anti-SCL70
B.   p-ANCA
C.   rheumatoid factor
D.   anti-glomerular basement membrane
E.   anti-Hu

22. A patient with a pneumonia has a small pleural effusion. Diagnostic aspiration is performed. Which result is most consistent with a malignant effusion

A.   low glucose
B.   positive rheumatoid factor
C.   blood stained fluid
D.   an exudate
E.   a transudate

23. A 35 year old recently returned from a Spanish holiday with loose stools and breathlessness. He is tachypnoeic at rest. CXR shows no focal consolidation.
The most appropriate investigation in this case is?

A.   V/Q scan
B.   CTPA
C.   HIV test
D.   urine legionella and pneumococcal tests
E.   blood culture

24. A 68 year old woman presents with small volume haemoptysis
She has a cavitating lesion in the right apex and a past history of TB in her youth.
The most likely diagnosis in this patient is?

A.   lung cancer
B.   reactivation of TB
C.   aspergillus

D.   PE
E.   Granulomatous disease with polyangiitis

25. A 70 year old woman with rheumatoid arthritis, treated with adalimumab, presents with a short history of breathlessness and has bilateral patchy consolidation on CXR. After initial treatment with antibiotics which is the most appropriate initial investigation to identify the diagnosis?

A.   bronchoscopy
B.   3 early morning sputums
C.   quantiferon test (interferon gamma spot test)
D.   Mantoux test
E.   sputum MC&S

26. A 49 year old man with a history of back pain for a number of years now has regular breathlessness walking up a hill while walking to work. He had asthma as a child and has not had any recent hospital admissions for asthma.
What is the most likely pattern on spirometry?

A.   FEV1 reduced, FVC reduced, ratio 0.8
B.   FEV1 reduced, FVC normal, ratio 0.7
C.   FEV1 reduced, FVC increased, ratio 0.6
D.   FEV1 reduced, FVC reduced, ratio 0.85
E.   FEV1 increased, FVC increased, ratio 0.85

27. A 20 year old with cystic fibrosis has recurrent pseudomonas chest infections. He is not improving following treatment with ceftazadine and gentamicin.
What organism may be responsible?

A.   Moraxella catarrhalis
B.   Pseudomonas aeruginosa
C.   Staphylococcus aureus
D.   Escherichia Coli
E.   Burkholderia Cepacia

28. A 65 year old man's spirometry readings are- FEV1 0.8 (30% predicted) and FVC 1.7 (58%). He is breathless on his current treatment. Based on the classification of his severity which is an appropriate combination of inhalers?

A. short acting beta agonist only
B. long acting beta agonist, short acting beta agonist
C. long acting beta agonist, long acting antimuscarinic, short acting beta agonist
D. long acting beta agonist, inhaled corticosteroid, long acting antimuscarinic, short acting beta agonist
E. long acting antimuscarinic, inhaled corticosteroid, short acting beta agonist

29. A 22 year old woman has frequent nocturnal symptoms attributed to her asthma. She is currently on a long acting beta agonist, inhaled corticosteroid and an as required inhaler. Her inhaler technique is good. What is the next step in managing the asthma?

A. add shortacting antimuscarinic
B. change long acting beta agonist to long acting antimuscarinic
C. add in long acting antimuscarinic
D. increase dose of steroid inhaler
E. short course oral steroids

30. A 34 year old man has deteriorated on the ward and you are asked to review him. He presented a few hours earlier through accident and emergency with difficulty in breathing. The patient has recently returned from a trip to South America. He was known to have severe asthma and was wheezy on presentation. He is alert but not able to speak more than 2-3 words and is pointing across his chest saying it is very tight. The nurses have him on a nebuliser and he is having 2 litres of oxygen to maintain saturations of 94%. ABG shows pH 7.41 PCO2 5 PO2 10 HCO3 24 & lactate 1.9
What is the next most appropriate action?

A.   treatment dose low molecular weight heparin and CTPA
B.   continue nebulisers
C.   ITU review
D.   IV aminophylline
E.   NIV

31. A 30 year old woman has had 1 teaspoon of haemoptysis. She is anxious about having a pulmonary embolus which her mother had died from after a hip replacement. She has had a productive cough with green sputum for 2 weeks and was feeling wheezy. There is no recent travel or history of respiratory illness in the past. On examination there are right sided crepitations with minimal wheeze. She is not breathless at rest or on limited observed exertion. Saturations 98% on air. Chest x ray showed a small area of right mid zone consolidation obscuring the right heart border. WCC 13. Curb score 0
What is the next appropriate step?

A.   anticoagulation and CTPA
B.   refer for bronchoscopy
C.   d-dimer
D.   treat with antibiotics
E.   anticoagulate and V/Q scan

2. Cardiology

32. 70 year old with a previous myocardial infarct presents feeling unwell. ECG shows a rate of 180 with broad complexes. He is pale and sweaty a BP of 70/50 what is the appropriate action?

A.   amiodarone
B.   adrenaline
C.   metoprolol
D.   DC cardioversion
E.   digoxin

33. 60 year old had a MI 3 days ago. He develops sudden onset shortness of breath. He is on a 15 L nonrebreathe and is tachypnoeic. There are bilateral crackles and a murmur. The cause of deterioration is?

A.   Dressler's syndrome
B.   pulmonary oedema
C.   ruptured chordae.
D.   ventricular septal rupture
E.   infective endocarditis

34. On the ward an ECG is done on a 60 year old man which shows left bundle branch block. The patient is having central chest pain. He is does not have any old ECGs on the ward. The appropriate action is?

A.   send off a troponin and then send a repeat in a few hours
B.   give aspirin, ticagrelor, fondaparinux, GTN and morphine
C.   refer the patient to the cardiology registrar for primary PCI
D.   request an echo
E.   give GTN and morphine

35. A patient reports chest pain which is central and radiates to his jaw. He has had a few episodes over the last few days which are worse than his usual angina pain. Examination normal, ECG sinus rhythm, no T wave changes, CXR normal, Troponin 6. The diagnosis is?

A. unstable angina
B. NSTEMI
C. non-cardiac chest pain
D. GORD
E. angina

36. A 19 year old person with bulaemia presents with a collapse at home. Serum K is 2.3. An ECG would show?

A. U waves
B. elevated J point
C. peaked P waves
D. peaked T waves
E. narrow QRS

37. A cardiac murmur is heard on examining a patient who has attended hospital twice before for pneumothoraces. The classical murmur in this case can be described as

A. early diastolic
B. mid diastolic
C. early systolic
D. mid systolic
E. pansystolic

38. Following a myocardial infarct discharge medications should include

A. aspirin, atorvastatin, bisoprolol, amiodarone
B. aspirin atorvastatin, atenolol, ticagrelor
C. aspirin, atorvastatin, bisoprolol , ticagrelor, amiodarone
D. aspirin, atorvastatin, bisoprolol , ticagrelor,
E. aspirin, warfarin, atorvastatin, bisoprolol , ticagrelor,

39. You attend a patient who has become short of breath. The nurses are just doing his observations. Saturations are 80% on air, RR 32, 120/85, HR 130, Temp 36.7C. He is speaking in one word answers. There are bilateral crepitations.
The first most appropriate action

A. ECG
B. CXR
C. Prescribe Frusemide IV 80mg
D. administer oxygen
E. call medical SpR for help

40. Of the following scenarios which one of them fits grade 3 of the New York Heart Association grading of heart failure?

A. breathless moving from one room to other
B. breathless walking upstairs
C. able to carry out light housework but gets breathless walking in the supermarket
D. occasional breathlessness on exertion
E. breathless when gardening

41. A patient presents with a BP of 180/120. Routine blood tests and urine dipstick are normal. There is no abnormality on fundoscopy.
The diagnosis is?

A. hypertensive crisis
B. accelerated phase hypertension
C. grade 2 hypertension
D. malignant hypertension
E. grade 3 hypertension

42. 39 year old with palpitations for 6 hours . Which is most likely to cardiovert him?

A. flecainide
B. bisoprolol
C. digoxin
D. sotalol
E. procainamide

43. A 80 year old woman has been short of breath for 5 weeks. She is waking at night and is sleeping on 4 pillows.
The single most likely diagnosis is?

A.   pulmonary embolus
B.   pleural effusions
C.   unstable angina
D.   pneumonia
E.   heart failure

44. There is T wave inversion in lead AVL. This is indicative of?

A.   myocardial ischaemia
B.   myocardial strain
C.   athlete's heart
D.   lead misplacement
E.   normal variant

45. 70 year old with bradycardia 40bpm who is well, normotensive and has an ECG showing complete heart block. Next most appropriate action is?

A.   atropine
B.   external pacing
C.   isoprenaline infusion
D.   cardiology review for pacemaker
E.   temporary pacemaker

46. A 90 year old comes in with shortness of breath and cough, CXR shows left sided consolidation. Heart rate is 110- 120. ECG AF. Blood pressure 89/50.
The most appropriate initial treatment with respect to AF is?

A.   digoxin
B.   bisoprolol
C.   amiodarone
D.   metoprolol
E.   IV fluids

47. A 25 year old with chest pain worse lying flat and eased leaning forward
Features on ECG include?

A.   ST elevation
B.   T wave inversion in inferior leads
C.   S1Q3T3
D.   sinus tachycardia
E.   anterior-lateral T wave inversion

48. Duke's criteria of endocarditis are met by which of the following?

A.   previous porcine aortic valve replacement, fevers, blood
      cultures x1 grow strep epidermidis, echo showing abscess
B.   Osler's nodes, blood culture grows streptococcus species x1
C.   Echo reveals tricuspid vegetations, blood cultures no growth,
      intravenous drug user,
D.   blood culture grows staphylococcus aureus x2
E.   fever, new murmur, echo shows vegetations on mitral valve

49. An 80 year old woman with a previous CVA and hypertension has AF.
Her CHA2DS2VASc score is?

A.   2
B.   3
C.   4
D.   5
E.   6

50. Blood cultures of a patient with endocarditis grow streptococcus bovis.
Further appropriate investigation should include?

A.   CT chest
B.   U/S liver
C.   U/S urinary tract
D.   colonoscopy
E.   sputum culture for AFBs

51. ST elevation in the leads II,III, AVF with associated reciprocal changes fits with infarction of which area?

A.   inferior
B.   anterior
C.   anterior-lateral
D.   anterior-apical
E.   posterior

52. A 60 year old with fast AF is shocked and sweaty. BP 70/40. The most appropriate action is?

A.   adrenaline
B.   DC cardioversion
C.   digoxin
D.   amiodarone
E.   metoprolol

53. A 39 year old man with chronic AF and no other comorbidities. What appropriate long-term treatment should he be advised to be on?

A.   none
B.   aspirin
C.   warfarin
D.   rivaroxaban
E.   anticoagulate for 6 months

54. A patient with an aortic valve replacement within the last year has vegetations on the valve. Which organism is most likely to be responsible?

A.   strep bovis
B.   staph aureus
C.   strep epidermidis
D.   strep pyogenes
E.   coxiella

55. A 60 year old woman, previously fit and well, presents with palpitations for 2 weeks. She is feeling hot and sweaty. She looks unwell. ECG shows atrial fibrillation with a fast ventricular rate of 160-170. Blood pressure is 125/75. TSH is <0.01. The most appropriate step is?

A.   rate control
B.   DC cardioversion
C.   assess for underlying infection
D.   discuss with endocrinology
E.   chemical cardioversion

56. A 60 year old man with no past medical history is brought in by ambulance with chest pain. It started after eating breakfast reading the newspaper. It is central and non-radiating. ECG shows no acute changes and the pain resolves with 1 spray of GTN. Troponin at 4 hours is negative. The likely diagnosis is?.

A.   unstable angina
B.   angina
C.   oesophageal spasm
D.   NSTEMI
E.   costochondritis

57. 80 year old man has presented with breathlessness with a chest x ray showing florid pulmonary oedema. He was treated and stabilised on diuretics.
Which of the following has not been shown to prolong survival in heart failure.

A.   carvedilol
B.   propranolol
C.   metoprolol
D.   bisoprolol
E.   nebivolol

58. A 70 year old with progressive breathlessness presents. There is a left ventricular heave on palpation and bibasal crepitations on auscultation. Which type of pulse is likely to be present?

A.   low volume
B.   collapsing
C.   normal
D.   bisferiens
E.   anacrotic

59. A patient has had a myocardial infarction with changes in II, III, AVF and deteriorates around 24hours later with hypotension and shock. Which of the following is most associated with the location of this infarct?

A.   first degree heart block
B.   atrial flutter
C.   atrial fibrillation
D.   bradycardia
E.   sinus tachycardia

3. Gastroenterology

60. 35 year old woman has had loose floating stools for 2-3 months and occasional abdominal discomfort. There has been no change in weight.
Her IgA level is low and anti-tissue transglutaminase is normal.
The next most appropriate step is?.

A. thyroid antibodies
B. OGD and biopsy
C. anti-gliadin antibodies
D. barium swallow
E. SeCAT study

61. A 39 year old has had reflux for several years that has been much improved by a proton pump inhibitor. There is a history of pain on swallowing for the last 3 weeks.
The next most appropriate step is?

A. wait for 2 week assess response to the proton pump inhibitor
B. OGD if there is weightloss or blood per rectum
C. OGD if there is anaemia
D. OGD
E. trail of antacids in addition to proton pump inhibitor

62. a patient with known ulcerative colitis develops deranged liver function tests. What autoantibody is classically associated with the underlying condition?

A. anti-nuclear
B. anti-microsomal
C. anti-mitochondrial
D. anti-smooth muscle
E. anti-LKM1

63. A 50 year old with known varices and alcoholic liver disease is admitted.with frank haematemesis As well as fluid resuscitation and blood products what additional treatment is recognised to improve survival?

A. terlipressin
B. vitamin K
C. platelets
D. colloid
E. antibiotics

64. A 24 year old man has had a decline in health over the last 3 months. He opens his bowel frequently and occasionally does so overnight. He has oral ulcers and a discharging sinus. Bowel histology would most likely show

A. rose thorn ulceration
B. predominant granulocyte infiltrate
C. predominant lymphocytic infiltrate
D. atrophic villi
E. transmural inflammation

65. A 50 year old alcoholic has presented with severe central abdominal pain. He is vomiting and unable to keep any food down. The single most appropriate initial investigation should include?

A. U/S abdomen
B. OGD
C. liver function tests
D. amylase
E. CT abdomen/pelvis

66. Liver disease runs in the family and they have been advised to avoid smoking as their health is put at greater risk. What condition do they have?

A. Wilson's
B. haemochromatosis
C. Gaucher's
D. polycystic liver disease
E. alpha-1 antitrypsin

67. A 40 year old man born in South East Asia presents with ascites and deranged liver function tests. He denies alcohol abuse. The most likely aetiology is?

A.   hepatitis A
B.   hepatitis B
C.   hepatitis C
D.   hepatitis D
E.   hepatitis E

68. A 70 year old presents with jaundice, weight loss and early satiety. There is no previous history of gallstones or liver disease. His abdomen is soft and non-tender. His bilirubin is 130, ALT 70 and ALP 400.
The most likely diagnosis is?

A.   pancreatic cancer
B.   gallstones
C.   alcoholic liver disease
D.   viral hepatitis
E.   a drug reaction

69. An immigrant is brought in by his relatives concerned about his general wellbeing. He has lived in a famine area for many years. They have noticed cognitive impairment, a skin rash and loose stool. These features classically occur in deficiency of?

A.   niacin
B.   thiamine
C.   pyridoxine
D.   vitamin E
E.   folic acid

70. 24 hours following an ERCP a patient has central abdominal pain and nausea. The abdomen is soft and there is no evidence of peritonism.
Which test will support the diagnosis?

A.   Full blood count
B.   LFTs
C.   amylase
D.   CT abdomen
E.   CRP

71. Which one of these is not a feature of decompensated liver disease?

A.   Jaundice
B.   confusion
C.   tremor
D.   ascites
E.   GI bleed

72. The following are triggers for decompensated liver disease. Which one is not?

A.   antibiotics
B.   GI bleed
C.   constipation
D.   hepatocellular carcinoma
E.   infection

73. Admission with jaundice and ascites triggers a review of a patient who has not attended liver clinic. Which one contains the routine elements of long-term monitoring care?

A.   u/s liver, OGD,
B.   CEA, AFP, OGD
C.   CEA
D.   u/s liver, OGD , colonoscopy,
E.   u/s liver, OGD, AFP

74. The gastroenterology registrar tells you that he has seen a rash under the armpits of a patient he has on the ward. A gastroscopy was performed the day before showing a suspicious gastric ulcer. What rash is likely to be present?

A. acanthosis nigricans
B. erythema ab igne
C. erythema multiforme
D. erythema marginatum
E. erythema nodosum

75, A patient with an oesophageal stricture has had an endoscopic dilation and is eating again. What abnormalities should you monitor for?

A. low phosphate
B. low potassium, high phosphate
C. low sodium
D. low magnesium
E. high blood sugars

76. In a patient with paracetamol overdose, which is not used as a criterion for considering an adult for liver transplant?

A. bilirubin
B. pH
C. creatinine
D. INR
E. encephalopathy

77. A 25 year old with ulcerative colitis is admitted through accident and emergency with increased stool frequency and blood PR. Initial observations – BP 100/70, HR 130, O2 sats 97% on room air, RR 20 /min, T 37.9C. Initial management should be?

A. IV fluids
B. Blood products
C. Abdominal X ray
D. Antibiotics
E. IV hydrocortisone

4. Endocrinology

78. A 60 year old woman has been admitted with a CURB 3 community acquired pneumonia. Her TSH is 0.05 (low) and FT4 8 (low).
The most likely diagnosis is?

A. primary hyperthyroidism
B. sick euthyroid
C. primary hypothyroidism
D. thyroiditis
E. euthyroid

79. A marathon runner collapses after the race. His serum sodium is 123, his serum osmolality is 285, and his urine osmolality is low. What is the likely diagnosis?

A. SIADH
B. salt losses
C. Primary polydipsia
D. cerebral salt wasting
E. diabetes insipidus

80. A 21 year old is admitted acutely unwell with the following blood gases- pH 7.05, pCO2 3.4, pO2 12, HCO3 11, BE -22, Lactate 2. These bloods gases show?

A. metabolic acidosis
B. metabolic alkalosis
C. metabolic acidosis with respiratory compensation
D. respiratory alkalosis with metabolic compensation
E. mixed respiratory metabolic acidosis

81. An oral GTT shows glucose at 0hr 5.8, and glucose at 2 hours 8.0. These results indicate?

A.   he is not diabetic
B.   impaired fasting glycaemia
C.   diabetes
D.   impaired glucose tolerance
E.   borderline result unclassified

82. A 55 year old diabetic with a recent MI has a HbA1c of 7.9. He is currently on metformin. What is the next most appropriate agent to add in?

A.   gliclazide
B.   pioglitazone
C.   linagliptin
D.   liraglutide
E.   insulin

83. You attend a patient who has a blood sugar of 3.0 mmol/L. He is sweaty but alert and speaking to you. What is the most appropriate action?

A.   glucogel
B.   IV 10% dextrose 500ml over 8 hours
C.   IV 10% dextrose 150ml over 10-15 minutes
D.   sandwich
E.   glucagon

84. A patient is reported by the nurses to have had a good urine output via his catheter. You review the fluid balance chart. He had a 300ml per hour urine output for the last 8 hours since midnight. He had been prescribed IV fluids containing 0.9% sodium chloride 1 litre 8 hourly and there is a prescription for another bag over the same rate. There is a history of head trauma 2 weeks earlier. What do you expect the results of biochemistry to show?

A.   sodium 159
B.   sodium 121
C.   sodium 135
D.   potassium 4.0
E.   calcium 2.05

85. A patient has a routine fasting blood sugar which is found to be elevated. He comes to see his GP. He has had no weight loss or polydipsia. He talks about his shoes not fitting and pins and needles in his right hand. He understands that he may need to start diabetic medication today. The most appropriate follow-up test is?

A.   repeat serum blood sugar in 4 weeks
B.   OGTT
C.   IGF-1
D.   HbA1c
E.   capillary blood sugar in clinic

86. A patient presents with vomiting and high blood sugars. Ketones are found on urine dipstick and blood gases show an acidosis. The severity of his condition is best indicated by?

A.   hyperglycaemia
B.   hypernatraemia
C.   renal impairment
D.   hypokalaemia
E.   hyperkalaemia

87. A 90-year old patient is admitted with lethargy and confusion. His serum sodium is 118 mmol/L. Which urine results supports a diagnosis of SIADH?

A. urine osmolality normal, urine sodium normal
B. urine osmolality high, urine sodium high
C. urine osmolality high, urine sodium low
D. urine osmolality low, urine sodium low
E. urine osmolality low, urine sodium normal

88. A patient is being managed for DKA. A repeat blood gas shows that things are improving. You are asked to prescribe the next bag of IV fluids (4th bag). The potassium on VBG is 4.0mmol/L. What is the most appropriate prescription?

A. 0.9% sodium chloride + potassium chloride 40mmol 1L over 6 hours
B. 0.9% sodium chloride 1L over 6 hours
C. Hartmann's solution 1L over 6 hours
D. 0.9% sodium chloride + potassium chloride 20mmol 1L over 6 hours
E. 5% glucose + potassium chloride 40mmol 1L over 6 hours

89. A 20 year old woman with type 1 diabetes is having 3-4 hypos a week having been previously been well controlled. On detailed questioning she vaguely reports being more tired recently. There are no other significant features in the history. The most appropriate investigation to confirm the underlying diagnosis is?

A. thyroid function tests
B. HbA1c
C. IGF-1
D. Synacthen test
E. serum C-peptide

90. A 70 year old man has a normal serum calcium and phosphate .
His Alkaline Phosphatase is high. His PSA is normal, and a
myeloma screen is negative.
What is the most likely diagnosis?

A.   osteoarthritis
B.   Paget's
C.   Rickets
D.   osteomalacia
E.   rheumatoid arthritis

91. A patient with marfanoid features, who has had medullary
carcinoma of the thyroid in the past, comes to clinic for review of his
scans. A lesion of which organ is indicative of a unifying diagnosis of
MEN2b?

A.   thyroid
B.   pituitary
C.   spleen
D.   adrenal
E.   parathyroid

92. A 20 year old presents with headache and drowsiness. She is
hypotensive and has a blood sugar of 3.5 mmol/L, a sodium of 121,
potassium is 6.6, urea 4.0 and creatinine is 60 umol/L. The
probable diagnosis is?

A.   SIADH
B.   adrenal insufficiency
C.   drug toxicity
D.   pituitary apoplexy
E.   cerebral salt wasting

93. These risk factors for osteoporosis are correct apart from?

A.   male sex
B.   female sex
C.   steroid use
D.   late onset menarche
E.   early menopause

94. A 60 year old man with type 2 diabetes controlled with metformin and gliclazide, has a Hba1c of 7.8, is admitted with a urinary tract infection. He is alert and talking to you. He is normotensive, tachycardic rate 110 and has a soft abdomen. Lactate on VBG is 4.5.
The most appropriate management with respect to his diabetes is ?

A.	stop metformin, add insulin
B.	start insulin and continue regular medications
C.	stop metformin, continue gliclazide monotherapy
D.	continue metformin and gliclazide but add linagliptin
E.	stop metformin, continue gliclazide and add linagliptin

95. A 30 year old man reports increasing pigmentation of the inside of his mouth together with 4kg of weight loss over the preceding 2 months.

The electrolyte abnormality most likely fitting this presentation is ?

A.	Hypokalaemia, hyponatraemia
B.	Hyperkalemia, hypernatraemia
C.	Hyperkalaemia, hyponatraemia
D.	Hypercalcaemia, hyponatraemia
E.	Hyperkalaemia, Hyponatraemia, hypercalcaemia

96. A neck lump is felt and investigated with a thyroid uptake scan. Sinister pathology is more likely with which pattern?

A.	cold nodule
B.	hot nodule
C.	diffuse generalised uptake
D.	generalised low uptake
E.	multiple zones of increased uptake

97. A 37 year old woman is referred from the urology department with urinary frequency. On detailed assessment she passes urine frequently and gets up to pass urine 3 times at night. She drinks 5-6 litres of fluid per day. She had a car accident 2 months ago which she mentions in passing.

The most likely diagnosis is?

A.   Transitional cell carcinoma
B.   Renal cell carcinoma
C.   Psychogenic polydipsia
D.   Diabetes insipidus
E.   Diabetes mellitus

98. A 75 year man presents with drowsiness, dehydration, calcium 4.0 parathyroid hormone level is low. What is the most appropriate initial management

A.   oral hydration
B.   IV fluids
C.   steroids
D.   IV bisphosphonate
E.   diuretic

99. A 75 year old with type 2 diabetes with blood sugar of 35 mmol/L, Na 156, K 5.9, urea 13 mmol/L and creatinine 190 umol/L. The initial management of this patient is?

A.   IV insulin sliding scale
B.   IV insulin fixed rate
C.   IV fluids
D.   s/c insulin
E.   insulin/dextrose, calcium gluconate

100. An 80 year old man walks in with an abnormally shaped head. His daughter reports that the deafness in his right ear is new. Treatment with which of the following medications will not alter his hearing but may help the pains he is experiencing in his leg bones?

A.   vitamin D
B.   bisphosphonate
C.   calcium
D.   teriparatide
E.   steroid

5. Geriatrics

101. A 65 year old present with a fall. He has had multiple falls and generalised weakness for the last 2 years. He has no tremor but has noticed wasting of the hand muscles. One of the diagnoses to consider is?

A.   subacute combined degeneration of the cord
B.   multi-infarct dementia
C.   Parkinson's disease
D.   motor neurone disease
E.   polyneuropathy

102. Classically, incontinence, gait instability and cognitive impairment are in keeping with a diagnosis of?

A.   dementia with Lewy bodies
B.   Shy-Drager syndrome
C.   multi-infarct vascular dementia
D.   chronic subdural
E.   normal pressure hydrocephalus

103. Prescribing in the elderly can be challenging. Which of the following medications does not prolong the QT interval?

A.   donepezil
B.   amitriptyline
C.   erythromycin
D.   bisoprolol
E.   citalopram

104. Dose reduction in the elderly is an important aspect of prescribing. Which of the following does not require a change of dose?

A.   benzodiazepines
B.   morphine
C.   haloperidol
D.   enoxaparin
E.   digoxin

105. Since this 85 year old lost his wife he is having difficulty remembering to eat and is having hallucinations of his wife sitting with him in the living room. What is the most likely diagnosis?

A.   vascular dementia
B.   Alzheimer's
C.   grief reaction
D.   schizophrenia
E.   space-occupying lesion

6. Rheumatology

106. A 65 year old woman presents with spontaneous right sided headaches which started the day before. She has some blurring of the vision of her right eye. There is no weakness of the limbs and her pupils are equal.
What is the initial investigation to confirm your suspicion?

A. CT head
B. MRI head with perfusion
C. ocular pressures
D. ESR
E. ocular CT

107. A 60 year old has had a few days history of a swollen and painful right knee following a return from Thailand. It is tender, swollen, and warm. The range of movement is reduced. He is afebrile. His WCC is 13 and CRP 40. The most appropriate next step is?

A. antibiotics
B. x ray the knee
C. serum urate
D. aspirate the joint
E. oral steroids

108. A 52 year old secretary has pain in both hands, particularly at the thumb bases
The most likely diagnosis is?

A. rheumatoid arthritis
B. psoriatic arthritis
C. gout
D. reactive arthritis
E. osteoarthritis

109. In the acute phase of SLE the results are likely to show?

A.   C6 C7 reduced
B.   C3 C4 reduced
C.   C3 C4 increased
D.   C1 reduced
E.   no change to complement factor levels

110. A 60 year old patient with haemochromatosis has pain and swelling of the left knee. Fluid aspirate microscopy is most likely to show?

A.   negatively birefringent crystals
B.   positively birefringent crystals
C.   cocci
D.   rods
E.   bacilli

111. A patient with rheumatoid arthritis who takes tablets and sub-cutaneous injections is admitted with pneumonia and has a neutrophil count of 0.4
Which is most likely the cause of the neutropaenia?

A.   rheumatoid arthritis
B.   sulphasalazine
C.   etanercept
D.   methotrexate
E.   leflunomide

112. A patient with painful muscles and a facial rash develops difficulty in swallowing. The clinical diagnosis is likely to be?

A.   SLE
B.   myasthenia gravis
C.   anaphylaxis
D.   statin-induced myositis
E.   dermatomyositis

7. Renal

113. Urine dipstick on a patient admitted with urosepsis shows leukocytes 3+, nitrites + protein 2+ blood 1+. The patient's WCC is 17, and creatinine 180.
What would you like to do confirm the diagnosis?

A.   send bloods for full vasculitis screen
B.   Ultrasound urinary tract
C.   CT KUB
D.   urine microscopy for casts
E.   IV fluids and antibiotics

114. A 21 year old man has noticed visible blood in his urine. He has had this a few times before following a respiratory tract infection. His creatinine is 80 umol/L. The most likely diagnosis is?

A.   post-streptococcal glomerulonephritis
B.   minimal change nephropathy
C.   membranous nephropathy
D.   IgA nephropathy
E.   lupus nephritis

115. A woman with chronic kidney disease for many years has the following results:
calcium 3.2 mmol/L phosphate 0.6, alkaline phosphatase is raised
The most likely diagnosis in this scenario is?

A.   vitamin D toxicity
B.   primary hyperparathyroidism
C.   secondary hyperparathyroidism
D.   tertiary hyperparathyroidism
E.   metastatic disease

116. A patient is admitted with sepsis and acute kidney injury stage 2.
The medications to withhold when writing the drug chart include?

A.   150mg ranitidine twice a day
B.   10mg ramipril once a day
C.   1.25mg bisoprolol once a day
D.   1mg warfarin once a day
E.   aspirin 75 mg once a day

117. A patient with pre-renal acute kidney injury has a potassium of 7 mmol/L on admission with peaked T waves on ECG. IV hydration and antibiotics have been started. What additional step would you like to take?

A.   calcium resonium
B.   salbutamol nebs
C.   50ml 10% calcium gluconate and insulin/dextrose 10 units in 50ml of 50%
D.   10ml 10% calcium gluconate and insulin/dextrose 10 units in 50ml of 50%
E.   IV sodium bicarbonate

118. A 40 year old patient who has had a renal transplant and is on combination immunosuppressant therapy is allergic to penicillin and is admitted with CURB 1 pneumonia. Which of the following would not be an appropriate antibiotic?

A.   doxycycline
B.   clarithromycin
C.   gentamicin
D.   vancomycin
E.   teicoplanin

119. The long-term management of diabetic renal disease with CKD involves medications to slow progression and prevent complications. Of the following which is of most benefit?

A.   furosemide
B.   metformin
C.   ramipril
D.   aspirin
E.   clopidogrel

8. Neurology

120. A patient with a history of alcoholism presents with confusion, ataxia and eye movement disturbance. The most likely diagnosis is?

A.　　posterior cerebral circulation infarct
B.　　anterior cerebral circulation infarct
C.　　drug toxicity
D.　　cerebral bleed
E.　　Wernicke's

121. A 29 year old has headaches which are throbbing in nature. He also has some visual symptoms which he reports as coloured lights. The history is most indicative of?

A.　　tension headache
B.　　subdural
C.　　migraine
D.　　glaucoma
E.　　cluster headache

122. A 90 year old presents with speech disturbance and left side weakness that resolved after 20 minutes. Blood pressure is 120/70. She has no past medical history. What is the ABCD2 score?

A.　　1
B.　　2
C.　　3
D.　　4
E.　　5

123. A 23 year old woman, who recently started the oral contraceptive pill, has developed a severe headache over the last 2 weeks that is stopping her from working and is much worse lying down and on waking up in the morning. What is the most likely diagnosis?

A.   migraine
B.   cluster headache
C.   tension headache
D.   cerebral venous sinus thrombosis
E.   subarachnoid bleed

124. Which of the following is not a core feature of Parkinson's disease?

A.   bradykinesia
B.   rigidity
C.   resting tremor
D.   impaired upward gaze
E.   freezing

125. Which feature of a tremor supports a cerebellar pathology?

A.   action
B.   resting
C.   improved with alcohol
D.   worsened by stress
E.   improves with chlordiazepoxide

126.The first presentation of an unprovoked uncomplicated seizure, pending specialist review, should have a minimum period off driving of?

A.   3 months
B.   6 months
C.   9 months
D.   12 months
E.   24 months

127. A 31 year old male presents with sudden onset of occipital headache associated with vomiting. There is no fever and bloods are normal. CT of his head shows no acute pathology. The next most appropriate action is?

A. Lumbar puncture
B. repeat CT head
C. CT head with contrast
D. cerebral angiogram
F. antibiotics

128. An 86 year old patient on the ward is noticed by a visiting relative to have developed speech disturbance over the last 5 minutes. On examination the patient has expressive dysphasia, a left facial droop, and left arm weakness. The first initial step is to?

A. contact stroke team
B. CT head
C. aspirin
D. thrombolysis
E. check bloods including clotting

129. A patient with macrocytosis and folate deficiency receives folate replacement from the GP and develops neurological signs. The condition present is?

A. myelitis
B. spinal cord compression
C. subacute combined degeneration of the cord
D. wernicke's
E. myeloma

130. A 78 year old presents with altered facial sensation. On detailed assessment there is right facial sensory disturbance, and left arm and left leg sensory disturbance. There is also some ataxia. The most likely diagnosis is?

A. lateral medullary syndrome
B. posterior cerebral stroke
C. Weber's syndrome
D. migraine
E. anterior cerebral stroke

131. A 37 year old has blurred vision on attempted adduction of the left eye and there is right sided nystagmus. This is indicative of a lesion in the medial longitudinal fasciculus.
This condition is most commonly associated with?

A. alcoholism
B. stroke
C. tumour
D. Wilson's
E. multiple sclerosis

132. A 32 year old woman has a dilated right pupil, poorly reactive to light, and it is difficult to elicit pupillary reflexes. The diagnosis is likely to be?

A. Holmes-Adie
B. Argyll Robertson
C. Weber's
D. central medullary syndrome
E. myasthenia

133. A 71 year old female with right ear pain and vesicles develops facial weakness on the same side. The diagnosis is?

A.   Lyme
B.   mononeuritis
C.   cholesteatoma
D.   Ramsay Hunt syndrome
E.   Bell's palsy

134. A 50 year old man with headache and eye watering. The diagnosis is?

A.   cluster headache
B.   trigeminal neuralgia
C.   migraine
D.   hemicrania occulta
E.   glaucoma

135. A 71 year old man has a painful right drooping eye with no history of trauma.
On assessment there is a complete 3rd nerve palsy. The most likely cause is?

A.   diabetes
B   hypertension
C.   posterior communicating artery aneurysm
D.   space occupying lesion
E.   cavernous sinus thrombosis

136. A 22 year old man with progressive distal weakness over the last 7 days has a lumbar puncture. CSF analysis shows a raised protein. The most likely diagnosis is ?

A.   transverse myelitis
B.   Pott's disease
C.   botulism
D.   tetanus
E.   Guillain-Barre

137. A 30 year old with a 2 day history of headache has a lumbar puncture. The CSF is predominantly lymphocytic. This result is in keeping with?

A.   TB meningitis
B.   viral meningitis
C.   bacterial meningitis
D.   subarachnoid bleed
E.   lymphoma

138. An 80 year old with progressive weakness resulting in impaired activities of daily living has noticed flickers of muscle movement and on examination there is wasting of the backs of the hands and brisk reflexes. The diagnosis is?

A. multiple sclerosis
B. metastatic disease of the spine
C. cervical spondylosis
D. motor neurone disease
E. diabetic amyotrophy

9. Haematology

139. Howell Jolly bodies are found on a blood film. The patient has which common condition?

A.   myelofibrosis
B.   lymphoma
C.   Diabetes
D.   Coeliac
E.   anaemia

140. Reed-Sternberg cells are found on the lymph node biopsy of a patient with recent weight loss. These cells are pathognomonic of which condition?

A.   mantle cell lymphoma
B.   Hodgkin's lymphoma
C.   diffuse large B cell lymphoma
D.   Burkitt's lymphoma
E.   T cell lymphoma

141. A patient with myeloma has blurred vision associated with hyperviscosity.
Which immunoglobulin subclass is most likely responsible?

A.   IgA
B.   IgD
C.   IgE
D.   IgG
E.   IgM

142. A patient with Burkitt's lymphoma has reduced urine output 2 days after starting chemotherapy. The most likely diagnosis is?

A.   tumour lysis syndrome
B.   hypercalcaemia
C.   renal stones
D.   haematuria
E.   outflow tract obstruction

143. A 50 year old with rheumatoid arthritis has progressive lethargy and haemoglobin of 80. MCV 85, folate and B12 are normal and ferritin mildly raised. The results are in keeping with?

A.   myelofibrosis
B.   Felty's syndrome
C.   methotrexate toxicity
D.   anaemia of chronic disease
E.   malignancy

144. An unprovoked DVT occurs in a 40 year old. Which of the following can cause thrombophilia?

A.   factor V deficiency
B.   VWF deficiency
C.   thrombin deficiency
D.   Christmas disease
E.   factor VIII deficiency

145. Following a single provoked lower leg DVT the minimum period of anticoagulation is?

A.   4 weeks
B.   6 weeks
C.   12 weeks
D.   6 months
E.   1 year

146. A 79 year old has bone pain, weight loss and a corrected calcium of 3.0 mmol/L. CXR showed multiple rib lucencies. The most likely diagnosis is?

A.   renal cell carcinoma
B.   lung cancer
C.   breast cancer
D.   lymphoma
E.   multiple myeloma

147. A 64 year old's blood results show low platelets, prolonged PTT and anaemia. This is indicative of?

A.   haemolysis
B.   disseminated intravascular coagulation
C.   an activated sample
D.   active bleeding
E.   haematological malignancy

148. A patient is blood group O. They can they receive blood from?

A.   group O
B.   group A
C.   group AB
D.   group B
E.   all

149. An 18 year old with a history of multiple hospital admissions presents with priapism. The likely underlying diagnosis is?

A.   thrombophilia
B.   trauma
C.   sickle cell
D.   recreational drug use
E.   medication related

150. An 80 year old who has a 4 weeks history of lethargy and some nose bleeds has the following on a full blood count- Hb 83, WCC 40, platelets 35.The likely diagnosis is?

A. chronic myeloid leukaemia
B. acute myeloid leukaemia
C. lymphoma
D. myeloma
E. myelofibrosis

151. A patient with known myeloma has increased lethargy over 4 weeks. His calcium is 3.2 mmol/L, and creatinine 140 umol/L (100). The most appropriate initial treatment is?

A. bisphosphonates
B. chemotherapy
C. steroids
D. IV fluids
E. diuretics

152. Acanthocytes are found on a blood film. This is in keeping with which condition?

A. iron deficiency anaemia
B. macrocytic anaemia
C. myelofibrosis
D. haemolytic anaemia
E. coeliac disease

153. A recent INR check for a patient on warfarin for atrial fibrillation shows an INR of 5 (target 2-3). The patient denies any bleeding. The most appropriate next step is?

A. vitamin K 0.5mg by mouth
B. vitamin K 5mg IV
C. omit a few doses of warfarin
D. reduce warfarin dose but continue
E. review other medications and continue at the same warfarin dose

154. A 70 year old man is due to undergo elective hip replacement in a few weeks. He has taken aspirin daily for 20 years following a myocardial infarct in his early fifties. It is felt that stopping aspirin outweighs the benefits in the perioperative period.
What is the most appropriate approach to advise about taking aspirin in this case?

A. stop the day before
B. stop 3 days before
C. stop 5 days before
D. stop 7 days before
E. stop 10 days before

155. A 85 year old man attends accident and emergency following an episode of slurred speech. He is on warfarin for atrial fibrillation and his INR his 8. CT head shows an acute subdural bleed without midline shift. Neurosurgical advice is for supportive management and to reverse the INR. The approach to reversing the INR is

A. fresh frozen plasma
B. IV vitamin K
C. omit warfarin
D. cryoprecipitate
E. prothombin complex concentrate

156. A 28 year old woman presents following a new DVT in her left leg which was unprovoked. She has had 5 previous miscarriages. Which of the following maybe the underlying diagnosis?

A. SLE
B. scleroderma
C. anti-phospholipid syndrome
D. protein C deficiency
E. polycythaemia

157. A 80 year old patient has a low haemoglobin, platelets and mild neutropaenia. Tear drop cells are present on a blood film. What is the most likely diagnosis?

A.   Felty's syndrome
B.   myelofibrosis
C.   chronic lymphocytic leukaemia
D.   coeliac disease
E.   folate deficiency

158. A 75 year old has recurrent chest infections. She has a longstanding history of rheumatoid arthritis and is on sulphasalazine. On examination her spleen is palpable. Full blood count shows neutropaenia. The most likely diagnosis is?

A.   methotrexate treatment
B.   Chronic Myeloid Leukaemia
C.   lymphoma
D.   Sjogren's
E.   Felty's syndrome.

10. Infectious diseases

159. A 20 year old presents with loss of consciousness witnessed by his friends. He remains drowsy and is being assessed for the intensive care unit. CT head shows ring enhancing lesions. Which test would be most informative if positive to understand the underlying diagnosis?

A.   Borrelia antibodies
B.   HIV serology
C.   CSF cytology
D.   hepatitis C
E.   blood film

160. A patient with sputum smear-positive pulmonary TB has started combination treatment. After starting treatment, when are they considered to no longer be infectious?

A.   1 day
B.   1 week
C.   2 week
D.   3 months
E.   6 months

161. A 62 year old patient with COPD has developed pneumonia. The genus of pathogen most likely to be causative is?

A.   Streptococcus
B.   Staphylococcus
C.   Moraxella
D.   Chlamydia
E.   Klebsiella

162. Which organism is responsible for slapped cheek syndrome?

A.   S. aureus
B.   S. epidermidis
C.   pox virus
D.   S. pyogenes
E.   rotavirus

163. A 17 year old with fever and a widespread maculopapular rash presents to Accident and Emergency. He has a sore throat and had been on holiday in Spain until a week ago. What is the most likely diagnosis?

A.   Malaria
B.   Leptospirosis
C.   allergic reaction
D.   HIV seroconversion
E.   Lyme disease

164. A man presents with vomiting following a Chinese take away at lunchtime .The vomiting started within 30 minutes of the meal. What is the most likely organism responsible?

A.   Salmonella enterica
B.   Campylobacter
C.   Bacillus Cereus
D.   rotavirus
E.   norovirus

165. A 30 year old Pakistani gentleman has developed severe upper back pain over the last 4 weeks. He has lost 3 kgs in weight over this period and has not been able to work in the retail shop in the last 3 days. A diagnosis to consider in this individual is?

A.   Pott's disease
B.   compression fracture
C.   disc herniation
D.   ankylosing spondylitis
E.   polymyalgia rheumatica

166. An 18 year old man returns from Malawi with a genital itch and an ulcer over his glans penis. The most likely diagnosis is?

A.   T. Pallidum
B.   H. Duceri
C.   Schistosomiasis
D.   Herpes virus
E.   Syphilis

167. An 18 year old presents with fever and neck stiffness. Which would be a relative contraindication to performing a lumbar puncture?

A.   platelet count of 50
B.   INR 3.0
C.   dilated ventricles on CT
D.   acute drop in GCS
E.   seizure within 30 minutes

168. An 80 year old living at home attends Accident and Emergency with diarrhea. There is a recent history of a UTI treated by the GP. The most likely diagnosis is?

A.   Salmonella
B.   C. Difficile
C.   Rotavirus
D.   Norovirus
E.   Campylobacter

11. Surgery

169. An 80 year old patient is catheterised for urinary retention. The residual volume is 1.5 litres. Over the first 2 hours he drains 400ml of urine per hour. You are asked to prescribe IV fluids for the patient. What approach is most appropriate?

A.   crystalloid 1 litre over 6 hours, then 8hr bag, then review
B.   match losses with IV fluids until the urine output slows
C.   prescribe 4 hourly bags, no faster, and reassess in 8 hours
D.   obtain an ECHO urgently to assist management
E.   stop IV fluids to reduce the urine output

170. A 77 year old man has a distended abdomen, diffusely tender with high pitched bowel sounds. Large bowel obstruction demonstrated on an AXR will show all of these features apart from?

A.   dilation greater than 8cm on the left side
B.   presence of haustra
C.   presence of valvulae conniventes
D.   bowel loops positioned peripherally
E.   no air in the rectum

171. Small bowel obstruction is diagnosed in a middle aged man with no previous comorbidity or surgery. The most common cause is?

A.   hernia
B.   adhesions
C.   constipation
D.   bezoar
E.   volvulus

172. A 76 year old has had a recent colectomy and end ileostomy for an obstructing tumour. The nurses ask you to review him as he has drained 30ml of urine in the last 6 hours and his blood pressure is 90/45
The most appropriate fluid prescription is?

A. crystalloid 1litre over 8hours
B. crystalloid 1litre over 4hours
C. crystalloid 500ml over 15mins
D. packed red cells 2 units
E. crystalloid 1 litre over 15mins

173. In the presence of tinnitus, vertigo and auricular fullness, the important diagnosis to consider is?

A. meningioma
B. Meniere's
C. cholesteatoma
D. labyrinthitis
E. benign positional vertigo

174. The initial management of an anal fissure involves all of the following apart from?

A. laxatives
B. local anaesthetic gel
C. seitan
D. diet modification
E. encourage hydration

175. A 32 year old man presents with left sided colicky abdominal pain loin to groin. Which is the most diagnostic test?

A. urine dip
B. u/s urinary tract
C. CT with contrast
D. CT without contrast
E. abdominal x ray

176. There is an 85 year old woman under your care for a community acquired pneumonia. She has a background of dementia and the nurse asks you to look at a rash on her right breast. What is the most likely pathology you will find in such a patient?

A. eczema
B. mastitis
C. allergic reaction
D. Paget's disease of the breast
E. cellulitis

177. A patient has undergone an elective laparoscopic cholecystectomy. Due to post-operative nausea the patient was not discharged on the day of the operation. The next morning the patient is haemodynamically stable but has had hiccups since 5am. What might you consider as the single most appropriate investigation?

A. U/S abdomen
B. CT abdomen/pelvis
C. CXR
D. laparoscopy
E. MRCP

178. A confused patient on the ward pulls out his urinary catheter with the balloon in place. He is now complaining of lower abdominal pain and has not passed urine for 6 hours. The most appropriate action is?

A. insert a 2 way catheter
B. insert a 3 way catheter
C. discuss with urology ? for suprapubic catheter
D. hydration and observe
E. abdominal CT

179. A 50 year old with a history of alcohol excess was recently discharged with severe abdominal pain that was managed supportively. He now presents 8 weeks later with nausea, early satiety and reduced oral intake. The most likely diagnosis is?

A.   pancreatitis
B.   pancreatic pseudocyst
C.   pancreatic malignancy
D.   GORD
E.   gastro-oesophageal stricture

180. A 65 year old is admitted with right upper quadrant pain. A diagnosis of cholecystitis is made. The patient is hypotensive, tachycardic, tachypnoeic and febrile. He has bloods taken and IV antibiotics and fluids are given.
Which of the following form part of the sepsis 7?

A.   lactate
B.   CRP
C.   LFTs
D.   calcitonin
E.   abdominal ultrasound

181. In the context of a splenectomy which vaccinations are important for the patient to have?

A.   hepatitis A
B.   meningitis C
C.   tetanus
D.   pneumococcus
E.   BCG

12. Oncology

182. 70 year small cell lung cancer has had progressive shortness of breath and facial swelling. He is unable to sleep on his usual 1 pillow at night.
The most likely diagnosis is?

A.   pulmonary embolus
B.   pneumonia
C.   unilateral pleural effusion
D.   bilateral pleural effusions
E.   SVC obstruction

183. A 78 year old patient presents with lethargy. Routine tests bloods and CXR are performed. His corrected calcium is 3.0 mmol/L and his CXR shows multiple round densities which the radiologist reports as cannonball.
The most probable diagnosis is?

A.   myeloma
B.   renal cell carcinoma
C.   lymphoma
D.   colorectal cancer
E.   thyroid carcinoma

184. The tumour marker associated with colorectal cancer is?

A.   CA125
B.   AFP
C.   CA19-9
D.   CEA
E.   HCG

13. Emergencies

185. You confirm a cardiac arrest and call for help. The correct chest compression to breaths ratio is?

A.   15:2
B.   30:2
C.   15:1
D.   30:1
E.   20:2

186. A needle stick injury occurs with someone who is known to have hepatitis B.
What is the risk of contracting hepatitis B?

A.   1/3000
B.   1/30000
C.   1/3
D.   1/30
E.   1/300

187. A patient on the ward being treated for a urine infection is known to have epilepsy. She is usually on levetiracetam and had her usual dose 2 hours earlier. You attend her with an ongoing seizure. The first appropriate agent to give is?

A.   lorazepam
B.   chlordiazepoxide
C.   phenytoin
D.   carbamazepine
E.   levetiracetam

188. A patient with bradycardia and hypotension has taken an overdose of propranolol. The antidote to this is?

A. hydrocortisone
B. adrenaline
C. glucagon
D. salbutamol
E. atropine

189. A patient is having a hypo and his blood sugar is 3.0 mmol/L. The medical registrar is on the phone with the nurse and she asks you to calculate the GCS of the patient. The patient is groaning, the eyes do not open with a sternal rub, and he can localise a painful stimulus. What is his GCS?

A. 5
B. 6
C. 7
D. 8
E. 10

190. The appropriate dose of adrenaline in a cardiac arrest situation is?

A. 0.5ml of 1 in 10000
B. 0.5ml of 1 in 1000
C. 10ml of 1 in 1000
D. 10ml of 1 in 10000
E. 10m of 1 in 100

191. In a cardiac arrest amiodarone is first given after which cycle?

A. 1st
B. 2nd
C. 3rd
D. 4th
E. 3rd and 4th

14. General practice

192. The first line antihypertensive for a 51 year old Afro-Caribbean is?

A.   doxazosin
B.   propranolol
C.   indapamide
D.   ramipril
E.   amlodipine

193. A 50 year old has a medical health check which showed a BP of 154/79. A repeat check at his GP surgery 2 weeks later found a BP of 150/79.
What is the most appropriate next step?

A.   start ramipril
B.   start amlodipine
C.   refer for ambulatory blood pressure monitoring
D.   recheck in 2 weeks if still elevated start medication
E.   recheck in 1 month if elevated refer for ambulatory blood pressure monitoring

194. A blistering rash on the elbows has developed in a 26 year old with loose stools. The likely skin condition is?

A.   psoriasis
B.   pemphigus vulgaris
C.   eczema
D.   dermatitis herpetiformis
E.   prurigo

195. An 80 year old with osteoarthritis of the knee has pain that is no longer controlled with paracetamol.
The next appropriate analgesic to try is?

A. co-codamol
B. tramadol
C. a topical non-steroidal
D. MST
E. buprenorphine

196. The INR is affected in the short term by co-prescription of which medication with warfarin?

A. penicillin V
B. clarithromycin
C. co-trimoxazole
D. trimethoprim
E. nitrofurantoin

197. A 67 year old man is hypertensive and overweight. His QRISK score is 12%.
What is the most appropriate action?

A. aspirin
B. beta blocker
C. clopidogrel
D. statin
E. warfarin

198. A 76 year old woman has had a new prescription medication recently that has caused dry mouth and blurred vision. Which of these medications is unlikely to be responsible?

A. oxybutynin
B. MST
C. amitriptyline
D. hydroxyzine
E. Indapamide

199. In an asymptomatic 80 year old man a routine blood test shows his sodium is 132 mmol/L and urea 8 with a creatinine of 140 umol/L (baseline 100). Which is the most likely medication that has been recently started by the patient?

A.   tamsulosin
B.   amitriptyline
C.   indapamide
D.   ramipril
E.   digoxin

200. The blood pressure of a 32 year old woman remains elevated 6 weeks after starting ramipril 5mg once a day. Routine blood test show sodium 135, potassium 2.8, urea 4, and creatinine 60.
What is the most likely diagnosis?

A.   a side effect of ramipril
B.   macroprolactinoma
C.   Conn's syndrome
D.   Cushing's
E.   Addison's

201. The blood pressure of a 60 year old type 2 diabetic is 160/85 on ramipril, indapamide, and amlodipine.
The next most appropriate step is?

A.   furosemide
B.   spironolactone
C.   refer to a hypertension clinic
D.   ACE receptor blockade
E.   refer to an endocrine clinic

15. Pathology, metabolic medicine and pharmacology

202. A 40 year old woman has taken an overdose 3 hours ago. She is nauseated, tachycardic, tachypnoeic and complaining of abdominal pain. The anion gap is normal and there is a respiratory alkalosis on her blood gases.
What is the likely medication she has taken an overdose with?

A.   lithium
B.   aspirin
C.   paracetamol
D.   sertraline
E.   citalopram

203. Kimmelstiel-Wilson nodules are associated with which organ and pathology?

A.   liver and cirrhosis
B.   prostate and hyperplasia
C.   liver and autoimmune hepatitis
D.   bone marrow and myelodysplasia
E.   kidney and diabetic renal disease

204. A patient with known myasthenia gravis has severe urosepsis. Which of the following is not appropriate in such patients?

A.   metronidazole
B.   co-amoxiclav
C.   vancomycin
D.   cefuroxime
E.   gentamicin

205. In the context of severe aortic stenosis, which of the following should be avoided?

A.   diltiazem
B.   propranolol
C.   GTN
D.   ramipril
E.   bendroflumethiazide

206. In the situation of a patient with a prolonged QT interval the avoidance of all medications apart from the following is appropriate?

A.   amitriptyline
B.   clarithromycin
C.   donepezil
D.   citalopram
E.   propranolol

207. Co-prescription of antihypertensive medications is common. Prescription of atenolol is to be avoided with which one of these?

A.   modified-release GTN
B.   amlodipine
C.   verapamil
D.   doxazosin
E.   digoxin

208. In the context of alcohol withdrawal, what medication is appropriate to prescribe to a patient being admitted with pneumonia who usually drinks half a bottle of spirit a day?

A.   lorazepam
B.   chlordiazepoxide
C.   methadone
D.   sertraline
E.   amitriptyline

209. A nurse has a few patients on medications with which she is not familiar. She asks you which one of these medications do not require drug level monitoring?

A.   lithium
B.   gentamicin
C.   levetiracetam
D.   aminophylline
E.   amikacin

210. Long-term side effects of amiodarone include all of these apart from?

A.   rash
B.   liver dysfunction
C.   hypothyroidism
D.   hyperthyroidism
E.   marrow dysfunction

211. A tablet controlled diabetic is having an elective laparoscopic cholecystectomy.
The most appropriate approach to diabetes management is?

A.   switch to sub-cutaneous insulin
B.   switch to IV insulin sliding scale
C.   hold off metformin but continue the others throughout
D.   hold off all diabetic medications on morning of the procedure
E.   continue all medications including on the morning of the procedure

212. The prescription of bupropion for smoking cessation should be avoided with which condition?

A.   COPD
B.   asthma
C.   migraine
D.   epilepsy
E.   depression

213. A patient has recently started a medication for seizures and now presents with a skin rash. The rash is likely to be?

A. erythema ab igne
B. granuloma annulare
C. erythema marginatum
D. erythema multiforme
E. erythema nodosum

214. A 35 year old with cerebral palsy and epilepsy presents with a chest infection and is not able to swallow any oral medication. The most appropriate management of his anti-epileptic medication is?

A. wait for swallowing to recover
B. convert to IV medication
C. insert NG tube
D. wait for a seizure
E. encourage liquid medication

215. A patient undergoing total thyroidectomy for thyroid carcinoma should be monitored for this associated complication?

A. hypocalcaemia
B. hypercalcaemia
C. hyponatraemia
D. bradycardia
E. seizures

216. A 55 year old woman presents with spontaneous lip, tongue and throat swelling a few days after starting a medication for blood pressure. Which is the most common drug associated with this condition?

A. ACEi
B. indapamide
C. doxazosin
D. bisoprolol
E. spironolactone

217. The toxicity of digoxin is enhanced by which of these?

A.   hyponatraemia
B.   hyperkalaemia
C.   hypokalaemia
D.   hypercalcaemia
E.   a beta blocker

218. A 40 year old with urosepsis is being treated with antibiotics. Blood culture results come back showing an ESBL producer. The patient is currently receiving IV coamoxiclav.
Which antibiotic will the organism be sensitive to?

A.   amoxicillin
B.   meropenem
C.   ceftriaxone
D.   cefuroxime
E.   penicillin

219. Zero order kinetics are a feature of?

A.   phenytoin
B.   propranolol
C.   rifampicin
D.   nitrates
E.   hydrocortisone

220. Besides chemotherapy the most common causative agent in drug-induced neutropaenia is?

A.   sulphasalazine
B.   carbimazole
C.   ramipril
D.   cimetidine
E.   aspirin

16. Answers and explanations

1. Centrally positioned lung cancers are most commonly small cell lung cancers. Adenocarcinomas are generally peripheral, and squamous cell carcinomas are central, but large bulky small cell carcinomas are characteristic and therefore the answer is small cell. **C**

2. The association of lung cancer with paraneoplasia is strongest for small lung cancers but based on frequency squamous cells cancers are more common and therefore cause more of this presentation in practice. **A**

3. A restrictive pattern should point you to pulmonary fibrosis. Anti-Jo is associated with dermatomyositis causing interstitial lung disease and therefore Gottron's papules is the answer. These are purple papules most commonly found on knuckles but can be on other bony prominences. **C**

4. An empyema is infected pleural fluid and diagnosed with a pH of less than 7.2. The other answers are pointing you in the direction of labelling the fluid as a transudate or exudate neither of which give you a diagnosis directly. **B**

5. Recent BIPAP indicated a type 2 respiratory failure. Target saturations should be 88-92% as the patient is oxygen-sensitive. Target Po2 is likely to be 8KPa in such a patient. **C**

6. Of these options there is only one that causes an exudate which is TB. Infection and neoplasia are the top two causes of an exudate. **A**

7. Knowledge of the British Thoracic Society guidelines is an important part of your revision for finals and day-to-day practice of a junior doctor. The next step in asthma management is adding inhaled long acting beta agonist. **C**

8. Nasal crusting and nose bleeds together with joint pains, particularly in this age group, is suggesting a multi-system pathology. The most likely is granulomatosis with polyangiitis (previously called Wegener's vasculitis). The distinctive radiological findings are nodules. The other findings are in keeping with dermatomyositis or polymyositis [for fibrosis], Effusions more commonly occur in SLE and RA. Hilar lymphadenopathy in lymphoma or sarcoid, and apical shadowing in ankylosing spondylitis. **C**

9. Extrinsic allergic alveolitis including silica exposure cause upper zone fibrosis. The other options cause lower zone pathology. **B**

10. Mantoux testing and TB elispot are not used in the diagnosis of active TB. It is a clinical, radiological and microbiological diagnosis. **B**

11. The top four options are all associated with cavitating pneumonias. M Cattarahlis is a pathogen associated with COPD exacerbations. **E**

12. There are classical findings on radiographs for PE that include options A, B, and D which are not common. An abnormal chest X ray does not rule out a PE and caution should be exercised in the context of these findings and investigating for a PE if the clinical picture fits. **E**

13. The interpretation of the blood gases should be systematic. Hypercapnia and acidosis are what you should look for from these options to give you your answer. Option C shows a metabolic acidosis, so the answer is B. Option D shows a chronic type 2 picture and this is compensated with elevated bicarbonate. **B**

14. There several relative contraindications which include most of the options. Invasive ventilation is preferable in pneumonia for respiratory support. The absolute contraindication and the odd one out is an un-drained pneumothorax which could develop into a tension one with NIV. **A**

15. A recent upper GI bleed precludes management with anticoagulation. The correct answer is an IVC filter. **D**

16. The most correct option here is type 2 respiratory failure (chronic). **C**

17. The most appropriate initial management is a nebuliser driven by oxygen as the patient is hypoxic. The patient should receive an hour of medical therapy before initiation of BIPAP if in decompensated type 2 respiratory failure. **A**

18. For some patients a V/Q can be appropriate. In this scenario with altered lung pathology CTPA is the most appropriate investigation. **B**

19. The patient has a significant pneumothorax without respiratory compromise. The management in this scenario according to British Thoracic Society guidelines is aspiration. **C**

20. All are life-threatening features apart from low Pco2. Normal or raised Pco2 in asthma is a life-threatening feature and it is important to recognise this and arrange an intensive care review. **C**

21. Pulmonary haemorrhage based on the clinical information occurs in either Granulomatosis with polyangiitis or Goodpasture's syndrome. C-ANCA is associated with the former and therefore the answer is **D**

22. Malignant effusions can have low glucoses and be blood stained but most are associated with exudates. **D**

23. In this scenario a hypoxic patient without risk factors for a pulmonary embolus with a recent history of holiday travel is suggestive of legionnaires since they may have had exposure to poorly maintained air-conditioning units. **D**

24. This is a classical history for an aspergilloma. **C**

25. In this scenario the patient could have a community acquired pneumonia and should receive treatment for this initially. The question is asking for you to appreciate that the diagnosis could be TB in the context of potent immunosuppression. For the diagnosis of TB in an unwell patient early morning sputums are of most benefit as they are less likely to tolerate a bronchoscopy. Quantiferon and Mantoux tests are not used in diagnosing active TB. **B**

26. This question has several parts. Firstly identify that the underlying diagnosis for the back pain that is being hinted at is ankylosing spondylitis. Secondly asthma is a distractor. Thirdly a restrictive pattern on spirometry is demonstrated in the last two options. Lung volumes will not be increased by a fibrotic condition which is present in this case. The answer is **D**

27. The most difficult to treat infections are in patients with cystic fibrosis patients **E**

28. This is severe COPD. Combination therapy with the full spectrum of agents should be given. **D**

29. Nocturnal symptoms are very important to enquire about in any asthmatic. Increased dose of inhaled steroid is the next step. **D**

30. Questions like this are not trying to catch you out with a change in diagnosis. It is given to you that the patient is being treated for asthma. With this in mind the patient is in extremis and therefore ITU review is the most appropriate step. **C**

31. Haemoptysis occurs in infection. The history of her mother is a distractor as it was a provoked PE. There is focal consolidation. A wedge infarct would generally not appear to obscure the right heart border. It is classically peripheral.

32. The management with any shocked patient with a tachyarrhythmia is DC cardioversion. **D**

33. The causes of decompensation post MI include reinfarction and arrhythmias but also structural compromise such as acute mitral regurgitation or ventricular septal rupture. A few days post MI, a murmur and pulmonary oedema, suggest that chordae rupture is the most likely diagnosis. **C**

34. New left bundle branch block with cardiac chest pain is an indication for primary percutaneous angiography. **C**

35. The history is very important in this scenario, particularly in terms of the quality of the pain and change from normal pattern. This is unstable angina. **A**

36. The characteristic features on the ECG are U waves and these necessitate intravenous potassium replacement. **A**

37. A patient who has had several previous pneumothoraces is likely to have an underlying condition. This would most likely include Marfan's or Ehlers-Danlos syndrome. The associated murmur would usually be that of aortic regurgitation which causes an early diastolic murmur. But an acute presentation with a murmur could represent an aortic dissection. **A**

38. The most correct answer in **D**

39. Correcting hypoxia is the first priority. Always remember ABC. Many SBA questions can be traced back to this principle. **D**

40. Breathlessness on minimal exertion is grade 3. **B**

41. In this scenario the patient is hypertensive without evidence of organ damage. The answer is **B**

42. The arrhythmias is likely to be AF. Flecainide is safe if the heart is structurally normal and is the answer. **A**

43. Progressive breathlessness and paroxysmal nocturnal dyspnea are suggestive of heart failure. **E**

44. This is a normal variant. **E**

45. In the case of a patient who is stable in complete heart block they should be placed on a cardiac monitor and observed. The use of atropine, isoprenaline or external pacing are used in the unstable patient and it is preferable for cardiologist to place a permanent pacemaker at the outset. **D**

46. In a septic patient with mild tachycardia in AF treating the underlying cause is the most appropriate action. The heart rate is being driven by the physiological stress response. Cardioversion may occur with amiodarone and the risk of stroke would need to be considered if the patient has been in persistent AF. **E**

47. The limited story is suggestive of pericarditis which is characterised by a saddle shaped ST elevation. **A**

48. Duke's criteria are a part of the last days revision before finals. The criteria are divided into major and minor criteria. **A**

49. The answer is **E**

50. This is a classical SBA question. Unusual bacteraemias are associated with colonic malignancy, and colonoscopy is the appropriate investigation. **D**

51. Knowledge of the coronary territories is important. Inferior - II, III, AVF; anterior/septal -V1-V4, lateral - V5-V6, I, AVL. **A**

52. DC cardioversion is the most appropriate action. If you are the first attender to the patient put out a periarrest call 2222. **B**

53. His CHAD2VASC score is 0. The answer is **A**

54. This is a common question. Staphylococcus and Streptococcus are the most common pathogens. Within the first year the exam answer is Strep. epidermidis. **C**

55. The initial management should be rate control. The TSH is suppressed so this is thyrotoxic storm and an endocrinologist should be involved as rate control medication alone is unlikely to be successful. Management may include carbimazole or propylthiouracil or Lugol's iodine. **D**

56. The history is suggestive of oesophageal spasm. **C**

57. This exam style question expects knowledge of the different beta blockers evidence base. The answer is propranolol. **B**

58. This patient has pressure overload with clinical signs of heart failure. The patient has aortic stenosis. The pulse to expect is low volume. **A**

---

59. The arrhythmia classically associated with inferior infarction is bradycardia. **D**

60. The history is suggestive of malabsorption. The IgA level is low which can give a false negative for anti-tissue transglutaminase. Further investigation should be an OGD and biopsy. **B**

61. Odynophagia is a red flag symptom and should prompt urgent 2 weeks referral for OGD. **D**

62. This is a factual recall question once you have identified that the associated condition is primary sclerosing cholangitis. The answer is anti-smooth muscle antibody. Anti-mitochondrial antibodies are found in primary biliary cirrhosis and anti-microsomal and anti-LKM1 in autoimmune hepatitis. Anti-LKM 1 is a anti-microsomal antibody. If there are two options where there is repetition of an answer with slight variation both are unlikely to be the correct answer. **D**

63. This is pure recall. The answer is antibiotics. **E**

64. The clinical history is suggestive of Crohn's disease as there are mouth and anal lesions. The histological pattern is transmural inflammation. Rose thorn ulceration is found in UC and inflammatory bowel disease will generally show a lymphocytic infiltrate. Atrophic villi are found in coeliac disease. **E**

65. The most likely diagnosis is pancreatitis whether acute or chronic. All the other investigations may be appropriate. An amylase is the single most appropriate initial investigation however. **D**

66. The answer to this question is alpha-1 antitrypsin. **E**

67. Chronic liver disease in South East Asia is prevalent secondary to hepatitis B infection. **B**

68. This presentation is due to pancreatic cancer. **A**

69. The triad of cognitive impairment, skin rash and bowel disturbance is caused by niacin deficiency which is dietary in origin. **A**

70. The differential of pain post ERCP is pancreatitis and perforation. In view of the examination findings amylase is the most appropriate investigation. **C**

71. The top four options are features of decompensated liver disease. GI bleed is a cause of decompensation. The other common causes of decompensation include infection and constipation. **E**

72. The only option listed that is not a trigger for decompensation is antibiotics. **A**

73. The routine assessment and monitoring of liver patients is to detect cirrhosis, varices and hepatocellular carcinoma and uses ultrasound, endoscopy and AFP. **E**

74. The range of dermatoses presented leave only one that is associated with solid malignancy. This has a leathery dark appearance, found in flexural areas, classically in the axilla. **A**

75. This question assesses your knowledge of the re-feeding syndrome. Electrolytes become low in response to the change in metabolism. Low phosphate is particularly of concern and is the answer here. Hypoglycaemia can occur as opposed to hyperglycemia. **A**

76. The criteria used in King's College Liver Unit to decide on transplantation include all the given options other than bilirubin. **A**

77. In such a scenario without more information such as haemoglobin or inflammatory markers, or stool culture, the initial management should always be ABC. The decision to give steroids should be after some stool results are back. **A**

78. Measuring thyroid function in acute illness will reveal suppression of TSH and cause this picture which is termed 'sick euthyroid'. **B**

79. In this case of hyponatraemia, where the serum osmolality is reduced and the urine osmolality is also low, water intoxication is the answer. **C**

80. This patient has a severe metabolic acidosis. Pco2 is reduced to compensate. The answer is **C**

81. This patient has impaired glucose tolerance the cutoff values are 7.7 and 11.1 for impaired fasting glucose and diabetes 2 hours after a glucose load. **D**

In a GTT impaired fasting glucose is 6.1-7.0 mmol/L; and in diabetes the criteria are fasting >7.0 with a 2 hour greater than 11.1

82. In the context of a recent MI insulin therapy is the most appropriate therapy to add in. **E**

83. In an alert patient the enteral route is the most appropriate and quick acting carbohydrate, glucogel, in this case is the correct answer followed by more complex slowly absorbed carbohydrate, eg cake/bread once the hypo is corrected. **A**

84. This question is testing that you can identify the connection between polyuria and head trauma and then what electrolyte disturbance is present. This is cranial diabetes insipidus and would correct with vasopressin treatment. As a junior doctor you are less likely to be called by a nurse to review such a patient as nurses may regard this as good urine output as they are more used to managing oliguria. A similar scenario, which is important to recognise on the wards, is post-retention diuresis. **A**

85. Different aspects of the history are needed to be fitted together. This is acromegaly. The patient has insulin resistance and carpal tunnel. The best test to confirm the diagnosis is IGF-1. **C**

86. The answer is hypokalaemia. This requires careful management in an HDU/ITU setting with central access as insulin therapy will cause translocation of potassium into cells lowering serum potassium. **D**

87. In SIADH there is inappropriately concentrated urine and the urine osmolality and sodium will both be high. **B**

88. Potassium should be replaced in every bag of IV fluids unless the potassium is climbing above 5.0. 0.9% sodium is the most appropriate crystalloid. **D**

89. The cause of hypoglycaemia in a type 1 diabetic is what is being tested in this question. The patient was previously well controlled. Without a significant change in diet, or insulin dose, or insulin overdose or change in exercise, none of which we are not told about, there is another cause and it is probably adrenal insufficiency. Synacthen test is the investigation most likely to assist in the diagnosis. **D**

90. With these results Paget's disease is the underlying diagnosis. Osteoarthritis and rheumatoid arthritis do not directly cause a raised ALP. Vitamin D deficiency will cause hypocalcaemia and if PTH had been measured it would be raised in vitamin D deficiency. **B**

91. The pattern of tumours in multiendocrine neoplasia needs revising shortly before the exam day. The answer is adrenal. To recap in MEN2b there is also a marfanoid habitus, phaechromocytoma and medullary carcinoma of the thyroid. **D**

92. A young person is presented here with hypoglycaemia, hyponatremia and hyperkalaemia. These features strongly suggest adrenal insufficiency but furthermore the patient is drowsy so this indicates that adrenal hypofunction is secondary to pituitary ACTH failure- pituitary apoplexy. Initial management includes steroid and crystalloid followed by brain imaging and neurosurgical input. **D**

93. Male sex is not a risk factor for osteoporosis. **A**

94. Lactic acidosis is associated with metformin and is associated with dehydration and renal impairment. Metformin should be stopped and most would discontinue it indefinitely. An additional agent is probably needed to control blood sugars and in this scenario insulin is probably the easiest. **A**

95. Increased pigmentation is caused by elevated levels of alpha-MSH which is co-secreted with ACTH. ACTH –MSH is very elevated in primary adrenal failure. This is (Addison's) and the characteristic electrolyte disturbance is the correct answer. **C**

96. A cold nodule is the most worrying result from an uptake scan. **A**

97. This young patient has polyuria and polydipsia following head trauma. There can be delay of some interval prior to presentation with the development of symptoms. **D**

98. The initial management of hypercalcaemia is hydration. With a raised calcium the patient is likely to need a bisphosphonate infusion but the initial management is with fluids. Many patients presenting with hypercalcaemia will have polyuria leading to acute kidney injuries as a result of volume depletion. Bisphosphonate alone would therefore be ineffective. The suppressed PTH indicates that the cause is likely to malignancy. **B**

99. The patient is hyperosmolar with a calculated osmolarity of 360. The initial management is with IV fluids alone until the blood sugar ceases to fall. **C**

100. A skull abnormality together with deafness in an elderly patient were classically described by Paget. The options presented are related to bones and vitamin D. The diagnosis is Paget's, managed with bisphosphonates, which improves symptoms. **B**

101. There is progressive weakness in this relatively young person. Particular mention is made of the wasting of hand muscles. This is more characteristic of motor neurone disease than subacute combined degeneration of the cord or polyneuropathy. **D**

102. This triad is a classical presentation of normal pressure hydrocephalus and a very common exam question. **E**

103. Factual recall. All of the options apart from bisoprolol cause QT prolongation. **D**

104. Caution in prescribing many medications in the elderly. Enoxaparin is not dose adjusted for age. **D**

105. There are several conditions which can appear similar to dementia. Grief reaction and depression are common pseudodementias. **C**

106. Giant cell arteritis is a common exam question and an ESR is the important investigation to send off. **D**

107. The diagnosis could be a reactive arthritis, gout or pseudogout. Joint aspiration is needed to rule out a septic arthritis. There should be a low threshold for aspirating a joint which is swollen and has a reduced range of movement. **D**

108. Thumb base pain is a common site for osteoarthritis and the occupation of secretary is a clue. Furthermore the isolated complaint is hand pain, particularly thumbs. **E**

109. Factual recall; the levels of C3,C4 are reduced in a flare of lupus. **B**

110. The association of haemochromatosis with pseudogout is being tested here. Pseudogout is caused by positively birefringent crystals which can be seen under polarised light and are rhomboid shaped. **B**

111. In patients with rheumatoid arthritis the most likely cause of neutropaenia is methotrexate. This patient is probably taking a biologic such as etanercept which is less associated with low white cells. **D**

112. Painful muscles and facial rash are not features of myasthenia. The diagnosis here is dermatomyositis. **E**

113. The questions tests how you assess the cause of an acute kidney injury. The most likely cause is pre-renal. The patient has uro-sepsis and the urine dip is only 1+blood. The kidneys leak some protein in AKI. Treatment of the sepsis is the most important principle in this case and the need to assess for the response. **E**

114. This a very common question. The answer is IgA nephropathy which has this characteristic story. **D**

115. The calcium is inappropriately raised in someone with chronic kidney disease. Therefore this is tertiary hyperparathyroidism. The patient has previously been hypocalcaemic due to impaired renal hydroxylation of vitamin D, which leads to subsequent excessive PTH production. **D**

116. ACE inhibitors should be withheld in the context of an acute kidney injury. **B**

117. The initial management of hyperkalaemia with ECG changes is calcium gluconate and insulin/dextrose in the doses given **D**

118. One of the most important drug interactions to remember is macrolides and immune-suppressants in transplant patients. **B**

119. ACE inhibitors together with managing hypertension and diabetes are core aspects of managing CKD. **C**

120. This triad is characteristic of Wernicke's which is due to vitamin B1 deficiency. Although a posterior stroke and drug toxicity can cause cerebellar features we are told the patient is an alcoholic and therefore the answer is Wernicke's. Treatment is with intravenous B vitamins. **E**

121. A young person presenting with these features has migraine with aura. **C**

122. The ABCD2 score in this patient is 4, due to age (1), unilateral weakness (2)
and duration being shorter than 1 hour (1). The patient is at high risk of stroke and requires admission for investigation and management. **D**

123. This patient has a postural headache which is worse lying down. We are told that she has recently started the contraceptive pill. Venous sinus thrombosis is associated with the pill and the answer is therefore **D**

124. The core features of Parkinson's disease are bradykinesia, rigidity and resting tremor. Freezing is associated with medication wearing off. The most correct answer- impaired upward gaze- is a distinguishing feature of progressive supranuclear palsy, a Parkinson's plus syndrome. **D**

125. The options present characteristics of different types of tremor. For cerebellar pathology the tremor is action. Two of the options are features of an essential tremor. **A**

126. Knowledge of the DVLA driving regulations in outline is important but always look up each case you are dealing with. In the case of a seizure, pending specialist assessment to risk stratify or diagnose, the period off driving is 6 months. **B**

127. Following a normal CT scan of the head the next appropriate step in management to exclude a subarachnoid bleed is a lumbar puncture to look for xanthochromia. **A**

128. The patient is FAST positive with a known time of onset. To allow rapid assessment and management contacting the stroke team urgently is the first step. **A**

129. This is classic sequence of events triggering subacute combined degeneration of the cord. B12 should be replaced prior to folate. **C**

130. This patient has crossed neurological signs. This is the lateral medullary syndrome. In Weber's syndrome the location of the pathology is in the midbrain with oculomotor palsy being a feature. **A**

131. This physical sign is inter-nuclear ophthalmoplegia. The location of the lesion is reported helpfully in the stem. This is most commonly associated with multiple sclerosis. **E**

132. Pupil variants or pathologies are common questions. The answer is a benign Holmes-Adie pupil. **A**

133. The eponymous syndrome in a list of options can often be the correct answer to the question. When there are two eponymous syndromes in the list this can be difficult. A Bell's palsy is generally said to be of idiopathic aetiology. Ramsay Hunt syndrome is reactivation of herpes zoster in the geniculate ganglion and is presented here with associated vesicles. **D**

134. Cluster headache is associated with autonomic features such as eye watering, nasal congestion and swelling around the eye. Symptoms last from minutes to a few hours. High flow oxygen can terminate an attack. **A**

135. All of the options cause third nerve palsies. A painful third nerve palsy is an aneurysm until proven otherwise. **C**

136. A distal progressive weakness in a young person with a raised CSF protein is likely to be Guillain-Barre. **E**

137. This question is straightforward. A lymphocyte-predominant CSF is likely to be viral. TB meningitis CSF initially has polymorphs but then becomes lymphocyte-predominant. There are no features in the stem to support anything other than viral meningitis as the diagnosis. **B**

138. The stem describes a mixed pattern of upper and lower motor neurone features. The diagnosis is likely to be Motor Neurone Disease. A structural cause should be excluded at first with cross-sectional imaging. **D**

139. Howell Jolly bodies are present in conditions in which hyposplenism is a feature. Coeliac disease is the only condition listed causing this. **D**

140. These cells with their typical nuclear appearance are characteristic of Hodgkin's lymphoma. **B**

141. Hyperviscosity is associated with the largest subclass which is IgM. **E**

142. Patients who undergo intensive chemotherapy with a high tumour burden are particularly at risk of tumour lysis syndrome which causes electrolyte disturbance and renal failure. **A**

143. This patient has a normocytic anaemia. Rheumatoid arthritis is commonly associated with anaemia of chronic disease. Be careful to note in an exam question that they are normocytic as a patient with microcytic anaemia could be bleeding from an ulcer secondary to non-steroidal medication. **D**

144. The only thrombophilia listed is **A**

145. If the DVT was unprovoked it would be 3 months. The answer is **B**

146. Bone and soft tissue abnormalities on chest X rays occasion themselves to present as myeloma. Always review chest X rays systematically. Of the cancers listed myeloma is the most associated with lytic lesions. **E**

147. Consumption of platelets and red cells is important to recognise and seek help in establishing a diagnosis. When reviewing blood results carefully consider the pattern of cell types which are affected. The answer is **B**

148. Blood group O is a universal donor and can only receive group O blood as they have antibodies to groups A and B. **A**

149. A young male who has multiple admissions has a chronic condition. With priapism as the presentation, sickle cell is the underlying diagnosis. **C**

150. This patient is anaemic with thrombocytopaenia and a raised white cell count. The likely aetiology is acute leukaemia. **B**

151. The initial management is IV fluids for all presentations of hypercalcaemia. **D**

152. Acanthocytes are disrupted red cells. Of the options given these are only present in haemolytic anaemia . **D**

153. Without bleeding a conservative approach is appropriate for a mildly elevated INR. With an INR less than 7 or 8 dose reduction would be the appropriate action. **D**

154. Aspirin is an irreversible inhibitor. The period off aspirin should be a minimum of 7 days. **D**

155. This patient has a significant bleed on warfarin. The INR needs to be reversed. Vitamin K is slow to act. Therefore prothombin complex concentrate is the correct answer. **E**

156. Several of these options are associated with thrombophilia. Anti-phospholipid syndrome is more associated with history of miscarriages in a young woman and is therefore the correct answer. **C**

157. A pancytopaenia can be caused by several of the options. Identifying the correct answer is dependent on making the connection with the blood film findings. Teardrop cells are found in myelofibrosis. **B**

158. Note the emphasis of the stem on 'longstanding'. The diagnosis is Felty's syndrome in which splenomegaly and neutropaenia occur in rheumatoid arthritis. **E**

159. A ring-enhancing lesion should trigger the differential of toxoplasmosis, lymphoma and abscess in your mind. An HIV test narrows the differential and is the answer. **B**

160. Factual recall: 2 weeks. **C**

161. The most common cause of pneumonia is Streptococcus. This is the same in COPD patients by frequency although the tone of the question might make one think of Moraxella which is associated with structural lung disease. **A**

162. Slapped cheek is caused by the pox virus. **C**

163. In a young patient with a maculo-papular rash and fever there are several differentials. These include measles and other common viral infections. In a patient with recent travel to Spain the stem is hinting at a different pathology and this is an HIV sero-conversion illness. **D**

164. This question is assessing the possible aetiology of vomiting. The incubation period is short and the patient has had Chinese food. The hint from the type of food is that rice has been eaten and this is associated with Bacillus Cereus. **C**

165. In a young patient with back pain and constitutional symptoms this is unlikely to be mechanical back pain. We are told he is of Pakistani origin. Pakistan has an increased incidence of tuberculosis. This is Pott's disease or TB of the spine. **A**

166. With a patient who has returned from Malawi the diagnosis is going to be water- related, schistosomiasis. This is a common exam question. **C**

167. All the options other than **A** are absolute contraindications, the others are relative. **A**

168. In an elderly patient with a history of recent antibiotic treatment the cause is going to be C. Difficile. Had the patient come from a nursing home with an outbreak of diarrhoea the answer would likely be Norovirus. **B**

169. This is post-retention diuresis. This can be a challenge to manage. Time will allow things to settle but in the interim maintain volume status as elderly men can easily decompensate with large losses. Match urine output with IV fluid input. **B**

170. The different features of small and large bowel obstruction are important to differentiate. Clinically vomiting is more likely to be present and at an earlier stage in small bowel obstruction. The options presented are features of large bowel obstruction other than **C**

171. The common aetiologies of small bowel obstruction are hernia and adhesions. This patient is young and has not had previous surgery. **A**

172. This patient is volume depleted with hypotension and oliguria. In this scenario the aetiology could be stoma related with high output or alternatively infective. The initial management should be a bolus of crystalloid. **C**

173. This is a classical history. The additional feature that could be included might be offensive auricular discharge. **C**

174. The initial management of fissures is supportive with analgesia and bowel optimisation. The answer is therefore **C**

175. A young patient presents with renal colic. The best test is a non-contrast CT because contrast will mask stones. **D**

176. It is important to have any appreciation of breast pathology as inpatients under other teams occasionally have breast problems. In this patient who has dementia there could be a medium to longstanding problem. Mastitis is most associated with lactation and allergic reaction and eczema are not that common and not generally localized in this area of the body. The answer is **D**

177. An awareness of the potential complications on the ward from different surgical procedures is important for junior doctors. Hiccups can be a significant symptom in surgical patients and it is important to obtain this history from the patient. The patient may not be forthcoming that it is a problem. It is a marker of diaphragmatic irritation. In the context of recent biliary surgery a bile leak with a sub-diaphragmatic collection is possible and cross sectional imaging is likely to be appropriate. **B**

178. This patient is in urinary retention and there is history of trauma. There may be history of haematuria with clots. This patient has clot retention and this is not an uncommon scenario to attend to as an overnight oncall FY1. The initial management is a three way catheter, bladder flushing and irrigation. **B**

179. Abdominal pain in an alcoholic needs carefully dissecting out. In the context that the patient has had a recent admission to hospital with abdominal pain this could be a recurrence of pancreatitis, alcoholic hepatitis, constipation, ascites, gastritis or oesophageal stricture. The symptoms reported are upper GI and with the recent admission referred to in the stem a pancreatic pseudocyst is likely to be the answer, if the original admission is presumed to be for pancreatitis. **B**

180. Factual recall; **A**

181. Asplenic patients are at risk from encapsulated organisms. The answer is **D**

182. Progressive breathlessness in a patient with lung cancer could include effusion, PE and infection. With facial swelling and positional breathlessness, the diagnosis to exclude is SVC obstruction. **E**

183. Hypercalcaemia and round densities on chest X ray are most associated with renal cell carcinoma. **B**

184. Factual recall; **D**

185. Factual recall; **B**

186. Factual recall; **C**

187. Seizure threshold is reduced in infection, fever and electrolyte disturbance. The initial management of seizure should be with benzodiazepines. **A**

188. Factual recall; **C**

189. Calculation of GCS is a common exam question and is important in day-to-day practice. A GCS of less than 8 means the airway is at risk and requires escalation to ITU and for an anaesthetist to assess the airway. **D**

190. Factual recall; **D**

191. Factual recall; **C**

192. Knowledge of a few NICE guidelines is important for medical finals. Guidelines to read are hypertension, heart failure and cancer referrals. **E**

193. This patient has two high blood pressure readings and he should be referred for ambulatory blood pressure monitoring to diagnose hypertension. **C**

194. A rash on the elbows with GI disturbance is characteristic of dermatitis herpetiformis. **D**

195. Managing osteoarthritis after paracetamol is no longer effective requires topical nonsteroidals and then escalation up the pain ladder. **C**

196. Learning the list of medications that interact with warfarin by P450 induction or inhibition is important preparation for the exam. In day-to-day practice, the interaction of macrolides with warfarin is one of the most important to be aware of. In view of the benefit of using the antibiotic it is often used with an increase in monitoring frequency of the INR and warfarin dose adjusted if needed. Ensure if you are discharging a patient on warfarin and clarithromycin to have a plan from your seniors and refer to the anticoagulation service informing them that you have given the patient an antibiotic which can interact. **B**

197. QRISK score more than 10% suggests that the patient would benefit from a statin. **D**

198. Medications often cause troublesome side effects to patients. Counseling is very important and it is important to engage appropriately with patients around adverse effects. All of the agents cause the symptoms given other than indapamide. **E**

199. The patient is most likely to have been started on an ACE inhibitor as indapamide mild diuretic. **D**

200. ACE inhibitors can cause hyperkalaemia rather than hypokalaemia. The answer is Conn's syndrome. **C**

201. The patient is on 3 agents for blood pressure. One last medication to add in is spironolactone according to NICE guidelines. Then the patient should be referred to a specialist clinic. **B**

202. The generalised symptoms of overdose which the patient has, are not discriminatory. Respiratory alkalosis in the early stage is suggestive of aspirin overdose. **B**

203. Factual recall; **E**

204. There are several medications that exacerbate myasthenia. It is important to look up and check when prescribing for these patients if a medication you are considering causes worsening of their neuromuscular problem. The answer is **E**

205. Factual recall; **C**

206. The answer is **E**

207. The co-prescription of multiple agents is part of routine practice to control blood pressure. Treating to target and avoiding symptomatic hypotension is the goal. The most noted combination to be avoided is calcium channel blockers and beta blockers and most notable, verapamil, can cause AV block. Diltiazem and amlodipine are considered preferable. **C**

208. The answer is **B**

209. The answer is **C**

210. Factual recall; **E**

211. For this scenario the answer is **D**

212. Factual recall; **D**

213. Factual recall; **D**

214. Epileptic medication doses should never be missed. An alternative route is always available. Seek help from a pharmacist or neurologist if there is uncertainty. The IV route in the short term is often the most straightforward. **B**

215. Thyroidectomy is associated with hypocalcaemia which can be severe. **A**

216. Factual recall; **A**

217. Factual recall; **C**

218. More and more patients are colonised with these strains of resistant organisms. There is only one suitable antibiotic from the list. **B**

219. Factual recall; **A**

220. The answer is **B**

Printed in Great Britain
by Amazon